Tinnitus No More

The Complete Guide on Tinnitus
Symptoms, Causes, Treatments, &
Natural Tinnitus Remedies to Get Rid
of Ringing in Ears Once and for All

Brian M. Lawrence
Copyright© 2014 by Brian M. Lawrence

Tinnitus No More

Publisher: Enlightened Publishing

ISBN-13: 978-1499127348

ISBN-10: 1499127340

Disclaimer

The Publisher has strived to be as accurate and complete as possible in the creation of this book. While all attempts have been made to verify information provided in this publication, the Publisher assumes no responsibility for errors, omissions, or contrary interpretation of the subject matter herein. Any perceived slights of specific persons, peoples, or organizations are unintentional.

This book is not intended for use as a source of legal, business, accounting or financial advice. All readers are advised to seek services of competent professionals in the legal, business, accounting, and finance fields.

The information in this book is not intended or implied to be a substitute for professional medical advice, diagnosis or treatment. All content contained in this book is for general information purposes only. Always consult your healthcare provider before carrying on any health program.

Table of Contents

Introduction

Tinnitus is sometimes called "ringing of the ears" and occurs when a sound is perceived by the ear with no external sound to go with it. Tinnitus is a common problem. Everyone has had episodes of brief or mild ringing in the ears but some people have it on a continual, chronic basis. It is estimated that about 10-15 percent of otherwise normal adults will have prolonged episodes of tinnitus that require a doctor's intervention or a natural remedy for the disease. Most people troubled with tinnitus are between 55 and 65 years of age.

As mentioned, tinnitus is common. When, in one study, participants were placed in an extremely quiet, anechoic room (without echoes), up to 93 percent of these people actually heard tinnitus even though they didn't complain of it under natural circumstances. These findings suggest that, in Western, industrialized countries, some damage because of noise is more common than most people think.

No one knows the exact cause of tinnitus. It is believed to be more of a symptom of another disease than an actual disease in and of itself. There are many causes of tinnitus, which will be discussed in later chapters. Tinnitus, fortunately, is not dangerous but it can cause impairment in hearing and is annoying enough to negatively affect a person's life.

People can develop tinnitus just by virtue of getting old as it can affect the aging ear. Certain medications can cause tinnitus to occur. The greatest cause, however, of tinnitus is excessive noise trauma to the ear.

The biggest problem with tinnitus is that it is completely subjective, meaning that only you can hear it. Others do not hear the sound and doctors often can't find any pathology in the ear to explain why you are hearing the unusual noise. Objective tests, such as audiometry testing, are often normal and don't help the doctor make any better decision about the diagnosis or treatment of the disease.

Some people experience tinnitus in just one ear, while others experience it in both ears. Most people say they have a "ringing" noise in the ear(s) but some people describe it as a whistling sound, a buzzing sound, a beeping

Chapter 1: A Crash Course on Our Hearing

There is one part of the ear that everyone sees. It is called the outer ear and is visible on everyone. It is connected to the middle ear through the external auditory canal with the tympanic membrane or "ear drum" separating the external auditory canal from the three bones in the middle ear. The small bones are designed to amplify sound so it can be heard easily by the inner ear. The three bones, also called ossicles, include the malleus, the incus and the stapes. Inside the inner ear is the cochlea, which takes "sound" and turns it into neurological signals that are picked up by the auditory nerve and sent to the brain for processing.

While the processes of taste, smell and vision have chemical reactions as part of their function, the act of hearing is purely mechanical. In this chapter, we will look at how mechanics plays a role in hearing and how sound from the external world reaches the brain in the interpretation of the sound.

Sound is produced when waves vibrate through matter, such as the air or through water. Air is not a void — it contains gaseous molecules that participate in the vibration that causes sound. If we breathed in a vacuum, sound would not be able to travel and we could not hear. Even solid objects vibrate when triggered to make sound. When, for example, you cause a bell to ring, you can see the vibration of the edges of the bell when it rings.

Sound is the process of "compression" when one particle collides with particles in front of it so that pushes sound forward. When the corresponding back flash of sound happens, the air pressure is decreased, resulting in a process known as "rarefaction". Sound, then is fluctuating air pressure — series of compression and rarefaction activities — that are picked up as differences in pitch. When the sound vibrates quickly, the pitch is much higher than when the sound vibrates slowly.

The normal ear needs to do three different things in order to "hear" sound. First, sound must be directed toward the part of the ear that hears. Next, fluctuation of air pressure must be sensed by the middle ear. Finally, the fluctuations must be turned directly into an electrical signal that is understood by the brain.

The outer ear or the "pinna" is what catches the sound waves coming from external places in the world. It has strategically placed curves that send the sound waves into the external auditory canal and to the middle ear. Without the external ear, we would not be able to hear as well as we can now. Because we have two ears, we are able to tell the difference between sound that is in front of us, sound that is to either side of us, and sound that is behind us.

When the sound wave travels into the external auditory canal, it directly hits the tympanic membrane. This is a very thin, cone shaped area of skin that is about 10.0 mm wide. It separates the external ear from the middle ear. Just inside the middle ear is the Eustachian tube—a direct connection between the middle ear and the back of the throat. When your ear "pops" it is because there was a difference in pressure between the middle ear and the outside air and the "pop" was the

Eustachian tube opening to equalize the pressure between the two areas.

The tympanic membrane is highly sensitive so that even the slightest pulse of air pressure fluctuation will cause it to move back and forth. It is kept tight by the action of the tensor tympani muscle, which allows the membrane to pick up tiny changes in pressure. Compression actions and rarefaction actions allow the tympanic membrane to move back and forth like a drum. The tympanic membrane moves more quickly when high sounds are directed to it and it moves over greater distances when loud sounds are directed to it.

The tympanic membrane is protective to the rest of the ear, particularly the inner ear, so that loud noises don't damage the ear. If there is a signal from the brain indicating the sound is too loud, there is a reflex in two muscles, the tensor tympani muscle and the small stapedius muscle, causing the ear drum to become rigid and less sensitive to the loudness of the sound. This phenomenon removes the input of loud and lower-pitched sounds so that the higher pitched sounds of conversation can be heard, regardless of the background noise. Interestingly, the same reflex is present when you speak out loud so that your own voice doesn't drown out exterior voices.

So how does sound get amplified so that it can be picked up by the inner ear? The compressions and rarefactions are really tiny and they need to be amplified before the inner ear can process them. The tiny bones of the ear, or the ossicles, are the body structures that amplify sound coming from the tympanic membrane and traveling to the inner ear. The sound waves not only vibrate the tympanic membrane but they cause tiny vibration movements of the malleus, incus and stapes (hammer, anvil and stirrup).

The malleus is located in the middle of the eardrum on the side considered to be the middle ear. This bone, in turn, vibrates the incus, which then vibrates the stapes that rests on the cochlea or inner ear by means of the oval window. The faceplate of the stapes presses inward on the cochlear fluid behind the oval window, creating larger than before waves that turn air pressure waves into water waves.

The waves are amplified because the surface area of the tympanic membrane is much greater than the surface of the faceplate of the stapes. This means a small sound on the tympanic membrane is translated into a much more magnified sound by the tiny stapes faceplate. The energy is concentrated in a smaller surface area so it is amplified. It also means that the pressure or force applied to the cochlear fluid is 22 times greater than the pressure felt at the eardrum.

Next comes the fluid wave in the inner ear. This happens in the cochlea that has the job of taking the fluid wave or "physical vibrations" and must turn that energy into electrical impulses that go to the brain.

What is the cochlea like? It contains three tubes that are connected to one another by extremely sensitive membranes. The tubes are curled up like a snail shell. Two of the tubes, the scala media and the scala vestibuli can be thought of as a single tube because the membrane between them is so thin that it doesn't really block sound waves.

When sound happens and the stapes vibrates, it creates a pressure wave throughout the cochlea. Inside the cochlea, there is a basilar membrane that is pushed in and out by the stapes. The wave moves across the basilar membrane to the other end of the cochlea. This basilar membrane is made of thousands of reed-like fibers. Some fibers—those near the oval window—are stiff and short, while others—those at the end of the cochlea—are longer and move more easily. What this means is that each type of fiber has a different resonant frequency that hums and vibrates at a different frequency.

Whenever the wave reaches fibers that have the same resonant frequency as the sound, the fibers vibrate intensely, like the strings of a piano. Higher pitches resonate near the oval window while lower pitched frequencies vibrate further down the basilar membrane (further down the cochlea).

There is a specialized organ called the Organ of Corti—a structure with thousands of small hair cells that lies on the surface of the basilar membrane and crosses the length of the cochlea. The basilar membrane moves wildly at the point that its resonant frequency is reached. The hair cells get activated at that spot and send a signal to the nerve telling the brain what was heard. The brain decides on the pitch of the sound based on which cells are sending the electrical impulse. If more hair cells are activated, the sound is perceived by the brain as being louder.

It's up to the brain to make sense of the electricity sent to it. The brain acts like a computer that interprets raw electrical data and can tell the difference between the same song played on a piano and one played with a guitar. Exactly how the brain does this is a subject of great research.

So now you know exactly how the ear works to hear sounds around us every day. What is more complex is why a person gets tinnitus—sounds that are perceived but are not really there for others to hear as well. We'll look later at some of the causes of tinnitus and some ways you can take care of the problem, especially using outstanding natural techniques.

Chapter 2: Understanding Tinnitus (Ringing in the Ears)

What is Tinnitus?

As mentioned in the introduction, tinnitus is when a person perceives sounds that are not heard by other people. It can be associated with loss of hearing, especially in the frequency range of the tinnitus sounds, narrowed blood vessels, ear tumors and other causes as listed below. Many hear the tinnitus as a high pitched whining sound, a humming sound, a clicking sound, or a whooshing sound. It is not only annoying; for some people it can be fairly debilitating.

There are many different causes of tinnitus. These include:

- Stroke
- Hearing Loss
- Loud noise exposure

- Wax or foreign body inside the ear canal
- Allergic reactions
- Medications
- Ruptured tympanic membrane
- Meniere's disease
- Ear infection
- Low blood pressure
- High blood pressure
- Fluid in the ear
- Neck or head injury
- Certain ear tumors
- Aneurysms near the ear
- Arteriosclerosis of the arteries near the ear
- Thyroid difficulties
- Diabetes

Uncommonly, you can get a temporary episode of tinnitus when loud noise exposure occurs. It usually lasts only a few minutes. If you get tinnitus that lasts longer than a day or so, see your doctor for an evaluation of the various causes of this symptom. Remember, tinnitus is a symptoms and not a disease in and of itself.

Symptoms of Tinnitus

Tinnitus is a phantom noise heard by an individual but not by others. It is heard as a ringing sound, a buzzing sound, a roaring sound, a clicking sound, a whistling sound, or a hissing sound. It can be soft or loud and, in pitch, it can be heard as a low roar, a medium tone or a high-pitched squealing sound. Both ears can be affected or just one. It can be perceived as loud enough to interfere with conversation or the hearing of external sounds. You can have it all the time, even when you're trying to sleep, or it can show up intermittently.

Types of Tinnitus

There are two major types of tinnitus: **objective** tinnitus and **subjective** tinnitus. Objective or pulsatile tinnitus is actually able to be heard by the doctor. The sound comes in pulses that match the heartbeat. The doctor can hear the sound by putting a stethoscope up near the ear, listening for what sounds like someone's pulse in the ear. It can be loud enough to drown out other sounds that might be heard. Fortunately, this is a type of tinnitus that only affects 3 percent of people with tinnitus.

Objective tinnitus is caused by muscular problems in the ear, problems with the blood vessels near the ear, Eustachian tube dysfunction, thyroid dysfunction and middle ear tumors. Objective tinnitus is usually considered a sign of a serious ear or other disease. People with objective tinnitus commonly have capillary malfunction near the ear, twisted arteries, high blood pressure, middle ear infection, neck tumors, inflammation of the middle ear, tumors of the veins (especially the jugular vein), and neck tumors. Ear wax buildup can cause objective tinnitus as can simple stress or depression. When the underlying problem is fixed, the tinnitus usually disappears.

Subjective tinnitus is by far more common than objective tinnitus, comprising 97 percent of cases. It is caused by abnormalities of the neurophysiologic system and, as such, can only be heard by the person experiencing the tinnitus. While it is not as serious as those who have objective tinnitus, it is still devastating to those who have it. It is stressful to experience and many people suffer from depression and anxiety because of their symptoms.

The major causes of tinnitus include loud noise exposure, old age changes to the ears, infections in the ears, some drug reactions, immune problems, poisoning with certain poisons, brain tumors, meningitis, ear drum problems, head injuries and toxicity. A condition called otosclerosis, which is a condition where bony growths develop in the middle ear, can cause subjective hearing loss. Even social and emotional problems like anger issues, hysterical reactions, grief/despair, anxiety, avoidance and fear can result in subjective hearing loss.

Interestingly, many people with subjective tinnitus can voluntarily modulate their tinnitus reactions. This allows doctors to help patients learn to control some of the tinnitus symptoms so the patients are more comfortable.

Risk Factors for Tinnitus

There are several risk factors doctors and patients must know about in order to reduce the chances that someone will get the disease of tinnitus. These risk factors include:

- Depression

- Increased stress
- Exposure at work or during leisure activities to loud sounds
- Tiredness
- Anxiousness
- Aspirin Use
- Quinine Medications
- Aminoglycoside Use (antibiotics)
- Diuretic Use
- Heavy Metal Toxicity
- Alcohol Toxicity
- Carbon Monoxide Poisoning

Diagnosing Tinnitus

When you see the doctor for your tinnitus, you will be asked about what your tinnitus sounds like and a medical history will be obtained. The doctor will do a complete exam, with special focus on a head, neck and ear examination. The doctor will ask about medication use and your exposure to toxins. He or she will also ask you whether the tinnitus changes with breathing and if you feel any dizziness or "vertigo".

Specifically, the doctor will use an otoscope, which is a magnifying device with a light that allows the doctor to look at the external auditory canal and the tympanic membrane. Fluid or inflammation of the middle ear can be seen using an otoscope. A thorough hearing test will also be performed and, in some cases, an MRI examination of the head and ears can be done to make sure there aren't any tumors causing the tinnitus.

Sometimes, patients with tinnitus are referred to a specialist in the disorder, called an otologist or otolaryngologist. There, specialized tests are done to see if there is a known cause for the tinnitus that can be corrected.

Tests for tinnitus include x-rays, an audiogram (hearing test), tinnitus pitch match, evoked response audiometry, tinnitus loudness match, maskability of tinnitus and residual inhibition testing. The x-rays may include a CT scan of the head or MRI of the head to look for tumors or vascular abnormalities.

The audiogram test will produce a chart that tells what the person hears at certain frequencies as well as the ability to hear speech sounds. Most people with tinnitus will have a degree of hearing loss, often at frequencies close to the tinnitus sounds they hear.

When the doctor uses evoked response audiometry, he or she suspects that the hearing problem and tinnitus is occurring in just one ear. It records inner ear sounds in each ear (neural impulses) as a result of sound provided to each ear.

In the tinnitus pitch match, the person is able to select from a wide range of audible frequencies in order to detect the pitch that the tinnitus is localized at. The pitch is measured in hertz. According to these types of studies, about 75 percent of individuals with tinnitus hear their tinnitus at a pitch match of more than 3500 Hz. This would be the equivalent of a very unpleasant, screeching sound.

In the tinnitus loudness match test, the patient is asked to listen to sounds of various loudness levels and is asked to match the loudness of the tinnitus to the loudness of an externally heard sound. Most tinnitus is heard between 4 and 7 decibels, which is barely above the threshold of actual hearing. This is unusual because most patients with tinnitus describe their tinnitus as being extremely loud when the studies show the actual sound is soft.

Sometimes a Visual Analog Scale is performed with a scale drawn from 0 to 10, with ten being the loudest tinnitus you can imagine. The person has to make a slash mark describing their level of tinnitus. When this test is done, 70 percent of individuals with tinnitus selected a value of six or more.

According to the Maskability of Tinnitus scale, the test measures the amount of sound it takes to mask the sound of the tinnitus. A band of noise is used from 2000 hertz through 12,000 hertz is sent through an earphone placed on the affected ear. The sound is increased until it is heard and then it is increased until the noise band masks the sound of the tinnitus. In most cases, the minimum masking level or MML is about 8 decibels or less. A few go as high as 22 hertz, but this is uncommon.

In the Residual Inhibition test, the amount of time the tinnitus is reduced or blocked within the ear after masking is measured. The test is usually performed by masking the tinnitus at about 10 decibels for one minute. After masking, the tinnitus is sometimes improved or disappears and this time is measured. On average, about 65 seconds of relief or improvement were experienced by sufferers of tinnitus. In several studies, it was found that increasing the masking decibels didn't do anything to change the degree of residual inhibition. Interestingly, the process of masking does seem to do a great deal to some people, who often get hours of relief after a masking episode.

Chapter 3: What Causes Tinnitus?

Tinnitus is commonly caused by damage to the inner ear. The small hair cells are normally triggered to send electrical signals to the brain when sound is appreciated. The brain then interprets these signals. If the hairs are bent or broken, the cells that operate them can send random signals to the brain in the absence of any noise.

Other common causes of tinnitus include other health problems related to the ears, certain chronic health conditions and injuries to the ear or brain that affect the hearing portions of your ears. Hearing gradually gets worse as a person ages, particularly beginning when the person is around 60. This hearing loss can trigger the presence of tinnitus in place of the lost hearing. This age-related hearing loss is called presbycusis.

Those who expose themselves to loud noises such as industrial machinery, chain saws, heavy equipment, firearms and other sources of chronic loud noise are at risk for hearing loss and tinnitus. Even those who play portable music devices like mp3 players expose themselves to levels of sound that can ultimately damage the inner ear hair cells. Even those who attend a loud concert can temporarily suffer from hearing loss and secondary tinnitus. Loud sounds over long periods have the effect, however, of permanently damaging the ears.

Earwax can block the external auditory canal. Earwax normally traps bacteria and dirt from getting near the ear drum. If the cerumen (earwax) becomes impacted, there is loss of hearing and irritation of the tympanic membrane, which can cause tinnitus.

If the bones of the middle ear become stiff in a condition called otosclerosis, your hearing can become affected and you can get tinnitus. This abnormal bone growth condition is hereditary so, if it runs in your family, know that you might get it, too.

Meniere's disease can cause hearing loss and tinnitus. This is a little known condition that is believed to be related to an abnormal amount of fluid in the inner ear or an abnormal pressure within the inner ear.

Stress, anxiety and depression can aggravate preexisting tinnitus and can cause it in some conditions. No one really knows how these emotional disorders cause a physical ear disorder but it appears that they can.

Temporomandibular joint syndrome or an abnormal TMJ, located on either side of your head and controlling your jaw movements, can cause tinnitus. People often hear a clicking sound or rubbing sound from the joint surfaces rubbing next to one another in an abnormal way. The sound travels through bone and is heard by the inner ear.

Neck injuries and head injuries can result in chronic tinnitus. Usually only one ear is affected because one side of the brain is affected. Similar to TMJ disease, neck injuries can result in sounds coming from bones that don't line up correctly anymore.

Some people can get a benign (non-cancerous) tumor of the acoustic nerve that causes sound signals to randomly be sent to the brain. This condition is also called a vestibular schwannoma and must be removed in order to have a chance that the tinnitus will disappear. Fortunately, it only affects the side of the head that has the neuroma and the other ear is unaffected.

Pulsatile tinnitus comes directly from blood vessel problems near the ear. The sound mimics the beat of the heart or is heard as a whooshing sound. There can be a head or neck cancer that presses on the blood vessels near your ear. The sounds coming from these abnormal blood vessels are picked up by the inner ear through passage through the tissues and bone.

Blood vessels blocked by atherosclerosis become stiffer and can't expand and contract with each heartbeat. The blood flow through these arteries is stronger and you can actually hear the sound of the blood flowing through these stiff arteries. The sound is often picked up by both ears because the problem is usually bilateral. The sound you hear becomes the tinnitus in your ears and is a problem usually found in the elderly.

High blood pressure or hypertension can cause increased blood pressure in the arteries near the ear and you can actually hear your pulse in your ear. Things like alcohol, caffeine, and stress can raise the blood pressure further and can increase sounds of tinnitus.

If a blood vessel is kinked in the neck, such as the carotid artery, or if a vein in the neck like the jugular vein is kinked, the end result would be turbulent flow through the vessels. You would hear the abnormal blood flow through the kinked artery to the ear and the result would be tinnitus.

You can have an arteriovenous malformation or AVM, which is a cluster of malformed capillaries that can cause an audible swooshing sound common in tinnitus. Because AVMs are rarely bilateral, you will usually hear such a sound only in one ear.

There are a number of medications used to treat various disorders that cause tinnitus or make it worse if you already have it. The more medication you take, the higher is the volume of the tinnitus. The various medications include the following:

- Cancer medications, such as mechlorethamine and vincristine

- Antibiotics, like chloramphenicol, erythromycin, gentamycin, vancomycin and bleomycin

- Quinine, a common medication for use in malaria

- Diuretics like Lasix (furosemide), ethacrynic acid, bumetanide and others

- Chloroquine, another malaria medication

- High dose aspirin, 12 regular tablets of ASA per day

Fortunately, when these medications are stopped, the tinnitus often goes away.

Chapter 4: Treating Tinnitus with Conventional Treatments

What can doctors do to treat tinnitus? Surprisingly, there are not a lot of traditional medical therapies for tinnitus, especially when the cause of the tinnitus is unknown. If there is a cause that can be found, sometimes all it takes is taking care of the underlying problem in order to take care of the noises you are hearing. When you know the cause of the tinnitus, a specialist can get involved in removing the acoustic neuroma, treating the TMJ disease or attempting to reverse arteriosclerosis.

Tinnitus, in some cases, can go away on its own. A person can have tinnitus for several months or years and then wake up one day without their symptoms. Another patient may be permanently disabled by their hearing problem and must live with it for the rest of their lives.

There are medications used to treat tinnitus. Some specialists recommend niacin as a treatment for tinnitus, even though there is scant evidence that niacin works to control tinnitus and it has several untoward side effects.

Neurontin or gabapentin has been studied by experts in the treatment of tinnitus. After high dose use, people were less annoyed by their level of tinnitus but the actual noise volume remained the same and it was not found to be better than taking a sugar pill.

Another study out of Brazil in 2005 utilized acamprosate or Campral. This is a medication commonly used to treat alcoholism. The study participants reported an 87 percent improvement on average. Studies have yet to be repeated in the US audience.

One needs to consider the cause of the tinnitus when looking at treatment. Some people can have tinnitus because of excessive earwax. Doctors can usually safely remove the earwax, decreasing or eliminating the tinnitus altogether.

If a medication is causing the tinnitus, the patient may do well to decrease the dosage of the medication or change to a medication that does not cause tinnitus. Vascular conditions can be treated with certain medications or surgery to the blood vessels can alter the blood flow so that the tinnitus decreases or disappears.

Non-medical choices for traditional therapy for tinnitus involve "white noise machines" or devices that mask or disguise the tinnitus sound. There are a lot of different white noise machines you can try to see if you find a frequency that decreases your ability to hear your tinnitus.

Other medications that have been tried in tinnitus including benzodiazepines, which control anxiety related to tinnitus, tricyclic antidepressants, which affect nerve signals, zinc, anticonvulsant medication, which affect nerve signals, and melatonin. As you'll see in the next chapter, there are many more home remedies and homeopathic treatments for tinnitus than there are traditional medical therapies.

Some patients respond nicely to cognitive behavioral therapy. This involves psychotherapy or talk therapy in which you learn coping strategies in overcoming tinnitus. It works well in some people and not at all in others. One generally talks to a therapist, a psychologist, a psychiatrist or a psychiatric social worker when dealing with these issues.

There is a specialized form of therapy called *"Tinnitus Retraining Therapy"* or TRT. It was invented by a doctor by the name of Pawel Jastreboff. Also called habituation-oriented therapy, it involves counseling sessions and audiological, tinnitus and hyperacusis evaluations. It involves painless electrical stimulation of the ear and has about an 80 percent success rate. The treatment works with the subcortical retraining of the brain so that it ignores the level of tinnitus. After retraining, there is a stage in which you are no longer annoyed by the tinnitus. You eventually get fewer and fewer periods of time where the tinnitus is perceived. In a sense, it is a process of habituation.

The tinnitus devices used are known as sound generators. They look a lot like hearing aids for both ears that mask the noise of tinnitus without interfering with one's ability to maintain a conversation. You can still concentrate on tasks and talk on the phone while wearing the device. It works for those who have hyperacusis as well as for those who have tinnitus. The devices are employed in order to increase one's ability to habituate to the tinnitus sound. Counseling is also used to complete the retraining process and is important to the success of retraining. TRT often takes 12-24 months to take effect but some people experience some relief after six months of retraining.

There are also tinnitus masking devices that are used to mask the sound of the tinnitus. They generate a low level sound so that the brain habituates to the sound of tinnitus. When you take the device off, the tinnitus gradually returns. These tinnitus masking devices create white noise that makes the noise of the tinnitus less (or resolved).

Some people need antidepressant or anti-anxiety medication because they have symptoms of insomnia or agitation because of the ongoing noises in their ears. Such medication can make the annoyance factor of the tinnitus much less; the patient is calmer and more collected around having this condition.

Some people use acoustic neural stimulation. It is a modern technique for those who have really loud tinnitus or recalcitrant tinnitus. It employs the use of a palm-sized device which is attached to headphones that give you a broadband acoustic signal that is embedded within music. It actually is felt to change the neural circuitry in the brain so you are eventually desensitized to the sounds of your tinnitus. It doesn't work in everyone but works in enough people to give it a try.

Some people use cochlear implants, especially if they also suffer from extreme hearing loss with their tinnitus. It basically bypasses the inner ear altogether and sends signals to the auditory nerve in the brain. It allows outside sounds to enter the implant, drowning out the tinnitus sound. The neural circuits of the brain are changed as it is in neural stimulation. In addition, your hearing will be vastly improved.

Because so few individuals suffer from known causes of tinnitus, medication to calm the patient, reduce depression along with masking devices are the best known medical treatments.

Chapter 5: Natural Remedies for Tinnitus Relief

Tinnitus has few traditional medical cures. This is in part because no one knows the cause of most cases of tinnitus. Rather than suffer unnecessarily, you need to know that there are many non-traditional, natural treatments for tinnitus that work just as well as doctors' treatments and tend to be much cheaper. In this chapter, we'll discuss the various natural remedies found to aid those who suffer from this annoying and frustrating disease.

The natural remedies are numerous. This is good because, if you find one therapy that doesn't work for you, you can switch to another therapy and will likely have good luck. Many of these treatments for tinnitus are inexpensive and have hundreds or thousands of years backing their claims. You can also try more than one remedy at a time.

Diets

Doctors and scientists believe there is a serious connection between what you eat and the symptoms of tinnitus. For example, you can hear unwanted sounds in the ear because of arteriosclerosis or possibly because of high blood pressure. Both of these conditions are diet related and are the result of a Westernized, bad diet. This is a diet high in red meat and other animal proteins, refined flour, refined sugar and processed foods that allow plaque to build up and stiffen the arteries.

Many others believe that a completely vegan diet will help cure tinnitus and there are those that have had good success with this plan. A vegan diet includes fresh fruits, fresh vegetables, whole grains and beans. It avoids all meats, eggs and dairy products. It is a diet that takes getting used to but is extremely healthy for you and reduces arteriosclerosis. It takes a few weeks of this kind of diet to notice a change so keep it up for at least that long.

Other types of diets that can make a difference include a three day fruit and/or vegetable juice fast. This can clear out earwax, which can cause tinnitus. Follow this up with a four week long course of garlic juice taken once daily. This will markedly lower the blood pressure and will dilate and relax the capillaries, especially when combined with a vegetarian whole food diet that is strong on a combination of raw fruits and vegetables. You should also take in virtually no saturated fat, including margarine and vegetable shortening. Your hearing and the sounds of tinnitus should drastically improve. Sugar is bad for you because it releases epinephrine in the adrenal glands, causing what's called "vasoconstriction" or poor blood flow near the ear. This, in turn, causes tinnitus.

Some recommend increasing the levels of dietary magnesium and potassium in the diet, including eating more baked potatoes, apricots, beets, nuts, leafy green vegetables or a multivitamin containing these minerals. Separate supplements of magnesium and potassium might be necessary in order to get enough of these minerals to affect a change in your tinnitus.

You also need to know that food allergies can cause tinnitus in sensitive people. The foods you need to avoid vary from person to person but it is a good idea to try cutting out dairy products, then grain products, then nuts, etc. Eventually, you may find a class of foods that don't agree with you and that stop your tinnitus when you stop eating them.

Cutting out caffeine, other stimulants, excess salt or quinine (such as in tonic water) might take care of that annoying tinnitus.

Some supplements may help those with tinnitus. These include the B complex vitamins, such as vitamin B12, vitamin B6, and vitamin B5 (also called pantothenic acid), which have been known to reduce tinnitus. People who take up to 50 milligrams of vitamin B6 two to three times a day have a reduction in the inner-ear fluid that then reduces tinnitus. You can also get vitamin B6 by eating bananas, whole grain foods, fruits, vegetables, dairy products and eggs.

There has been research showing a high incidence of tinnitus in people who are vitamin B12 deficient. Those people were also often exposed to a great deal of industrial noise. These types of people were then given vitamin B12 injections and had a reduction in their level of tinnitus. A person can take oral B12 as well even though this is less well studied. Nutritionists in general recommend that you take a supplement containing 6 micrograms of vitamin B12 every day. Common sources of vitamin B12 include oysters, milk, milk products, eggs, lamb, fish and poultry.

Vitamin A deficiency is known to cause problems with ringing in the ears and is a vitamin normally required for the creation of the ear membranes. You can get more vitamin A in your diet through eating oily fish, blueberries, dark green leafy vegetables (carrots and yams), and fruits (oranges, apricots and cantaloupe). Taking vitamin A supplements at 5000-10,000 IU per day can also be effective against tinnitus.

Vitamin E is helpful against tinnitus because it improves oxygenation of the cells and is an anti-oxidant. You can find vitamin E by eating more dried beans, leafy green vegetables, fish, eggs and whole grain products.

Choline has been known to clear tinnitus in some people after taking it for less than 2 weeks. It works best in those who have high blood pressure as a cause of their tinnitus. Choline can be gotten through taking two lecithin capsules with each meal (three times a day) or by taking two tablespoons of Brewer's yeast every day.

High doses of zinc have been found to help reduce tinnitus in the elderly. Some people have had complete resolution of their tinnitus.

Some have been known to have low zinc levels from the beginning; these people benefit the most from zinc supplementation. Some degree of improvement was found in 25 percent of those people who took zinc for a total of three to six months. The recommended dose of zinc is no more than 80 milligrams per day unless your doctor approves a higher dose. Foods that contain zinc are fish, beans, nuts, eggs, whole grain cereals and oysters.

Fresh pineapple has been known to reduce the incidence of buzzing and ringing in the ears from tinnitus. Vitamin C is found in high doses in pineapple and this is a strong antioxidant vitamin. Pineapple also contains bromelain, which is an enzyme that has promise in reducing inflammation of the inner ear. Fresh pineapple is most appropriate because cooking or freezing pineapple can destroy too much of the bromelain.

Why try lean proteins? Because these are the body's building blocks and are necessary for healthy brain growth and inner ear function. When thinking of eating lean protein, stick to tofu, legumes, seeds, nuts, and white-meat poultry. Red meats and dark chicken meat are not appropriate choices because they are high in saturated fats, which can increase earwax production and can worsen tinnitus.

How can you put this together with a diet that will reduce your tinnitus for good? Try a sampling of the above foods, choosing at least one food from each vitamin or mineral. Then make sure you include plenty of fresh pineapple, kelp, sea vegetables and garlic. Cut back on sugar, caffeine, alcohol, sodium and chocolate. There is some evidence that foods high in antioxidants, such as whole grains, fruits and vegetables can improve your hearing and reduce tinnitus.

There are several nutritional supplements you'll want to include as part of a healthy diet. Many of these will be discussed further in the chapter, in the section entitled "Herbal Remedies". These include Gingko biloba, coenzyme A, coenzyme Q10, vitamin C with bioflavanoids, B complex vitamins, vitamin E, hyssop, eucalyptus, mullein, and thyme. Some have been studied more extensively than others in scientific research studies on tinnitus.

Exercise Therapy

There have been various exercises and activities that have been known to relieve the symptoms of tinnitus. One ancient remedy involving exercise is called Qigong (pronounced "chee-gung"). It is an ancient form of Chinese exercise that is at least 2500 years of age. Some research indicates that it is at least 5000 years old. While the practice is ancient, at least one recent study showed that qigong reduced the symptoms of tinnitus in those who suffered from it. It is possible that qigong stimulates the auditory nervous system; however, more research is necessary in order to find out exactly how this form of therapy works.

Qigong is a form of healing and energy medicine. It uses specific breathing techniques, along with gentle and purposeful movement, and the art of meditation in order to strengthen the body's life energy and to cleanse and circulate life energy. Your mind is at peace after a qigong activity and you feel calm and tranquil.

Tai Chi can also be referred to as Taiji Quan. It is a specialized form of Qigong. It involves slow and graceful movements that look as though you are dancing. Qigong, as a whole, can be targeted toward things like tinnitus or other nervous system or endocrine problem; however Tai Chi acts on the whole body and mind. It attempts to restore the body as a whole by doing measured, slow and graceful movements along with careful breathing techniques.

Qigong involves four major areas of application. The one used most in the treatment of tinnitus includes Yi Gong, which is also called healing qigong. It involves preventative and self-healing techniques that reduce stress and control issues like tinnitus, high blood pressure, anxiety and frustration. You maintain a positive presence with qigong.

External qigong involves a having healer tap into healing energy that exists in nature and place it into their body, helping you heal. There are massage techniques, breathing techniques, and meditation exercises that go along with external qigong and some use therapeutic touch, deep massage, and acupuncture to help tinnitus heal itself. For a more Western touch, this form of therapy can be used with psychological therapies for tinnitus.

The two other areas of qigong used to manage certain conditions include sports-related qigong, which improves flexibility, balance, speed, coordination, strength, and stamina for those interested in sports and spiritual qigong. This helps people improve their self-awareness, harmony with nature and overall tranquility. It is related to the religions of Taoism and Buddhism.

Qigong does not have to be practiced by the physically healthy and can help people with tinnitus who are older, wheelchair bound or even supine. It can always be tailored to manage those who have mobility problems. Experts feel that it can be safely used along with traditional medications and therapies in the management of tinnitus.

Some people can get relief of tinnitus using jaw exercises. People use jaw exercises to increase the ability of the jaw to be flexible.

- For the first exercise, you need to open your mouth just slightly while putting two fingers upon the lower front teeth. Widen your mouth slowly as wide as you find comfortable.

- In the second exercise, you open your mouth against resistance, by holding the chin in the palm of your hand.

- In the third exercise, bite down while looking at the two front teeth. Then gradually open your mouth.

- In the fourth exercise, you need to open your jaw about one inch wide. Shift the jaw from left to center and from right to center. Repeat this ten times.

In fact you need to repeat each exercise ten times and do them at least once per day. After several weeks, you jaw will be more flexible, will click less often and you should have a reduction in your tinnitus, particularly if it was related to your jaw.

Yoga can do wonders for tinnitus. The breathing exercises of yoga can help regulate the inside and outside pressure of the tympanic membrane. The yoga pose that works the best for tinnitus involves lying in a comfortable position, with your arms at your sides or across your belly. You need to close your eyes and breathe through your nose deeply. Hold the breath in for one to two seconds, pushing the breath in through your stomach area instead of your chest. Exhale through your mouth, thoroughly letting the breath out completely. In order to treat tinnitus, you should practice this yoga breathing technique twice a day, 5-10 minutes at a time, for several weeks

Regular exercise of just about any kind can help reduce the symptoms of tinnitus. Exercise clears your body of toxins that can affect the circulation of the ears. It can decrease the noise you hear in tinnitus and it can reduce the number of episodes of tinnitus that you get. Exercises such as jogging, walking, biking, dancing, swimming, and martial arts are all great exercise types that can reduce the incidence of tinnitus. You need to be moderate in your activity because intense activity for long periods of time has a way of increasing the symptoms of tinnitus. If you have any questions about what kinds of activities to do and at what rate, talk to your doctor beforehand.

Because tinnitus is caused by several different possible things, exercise won't always help and certain exercises will help more than others. You need different strategies to take care of tinnitus of different causes so trying different exercise programs is a good idea. In general, exercise improves blood flow to the ear structures, which reduces tinnitus. Choose an exercise type that you like and can do easily so that you can reduce your tinnitus with something you enjoy doing. Increasing your level of activity should also lower your blood pressure, which can reduce the symptoms of tinnitus.

Avoid exercises that are noisier such as motorbike riding or skydiving. These can make tinnitus worse. Instead choose a regular form of exercise that doesn't overstress your system and that isn't too boring. Exercise you are willing to do on a daily or near-daily basis is the best one for your tinnitus. Ask your doctor if you are physically capable of doing the form of exercise that you propose. Then get the right clothing and gear; get professional instruction in the form of exercise you are proposing and get an exercise partner if that will help you get out there and do something that will stimulate your body to move.

Herbal Remedies

There are numerous herbal remedies for the treatment of tinnitus. Some have been studied better than others. There is no money in studying herbal remedies for any type of illness so most research is done by universities rather than pharmaceutical companies. Much of the herbal treatment for tinnitus is based on the extensive knowledge and experience of herbalists who have treated those with tinnitus in the past.

Gingko biloba is an herbal remedy that has been in use in ancient Chinese medicine dating back 5,000 years or so. It is known to increase the blood flow to the brain and inner ear, therefore decreasing the sensations of tinnitus. Gingko biloba is one of the most popular and most effective herbs for tinnitus, mostly due to its effect on brain circulation. Gingko has been known to reverse the signs of aging, making it especially good for age-related tinnitus. Ask your favorite herbalist about the dosage for gingko biloba.

Black cohosh has several uses; the most commonly known one is for female menopause. For tinnitus, however, it works wonders because it improves the blood flow to the brain which enhances neural connections. It is also a purely natural sedative so you won't be as stressed out about the sounds you hear.

Mullein is a diuretic that, combined with a low sodium diet, keeps fluid out of your system and especially from building up too much in your inner ear. This secondarily decreases tinnitus.

Some people can get tinnitus just by having high blood pressure. This means that rosemary is a good choice for those that have tinnitus because of their high blood pressure. It dilates the blood vessels to allow better blood flow to the ears, makes blood pressure more stable, and helps the inner ear function better as a result. Rosemary carries the official name of Rosmarinus officinale. It also invigorates the body, helping promote a more balanced mood with extra energy and zeal for life.

The herb known as avena sativa is better known to lay people as "wild oats". By reducing cholesterol, it prevents hardening of the arteries, improves circulation and therefore helps tinnitus. It is also a restorative herb and a tonic for nerves that need help, such as in tinnitus. Your energy level will improve as well when taking avena sativa.

The combination of Chinese yam, Chinese foxglove and cornus, made by a skilled herbalist can have a tremendously good effect in relieving the symptoms of tinnitus. They must be taken together in order to have an effect on the disorder. By treating your tinnitus, it helps you with your overall health and wellness.

There is an herb known as Verbena offici-nalis, which has special properties of relieving stress and tension, two known causes of wors-ened tinnitus. It promotes harmony and bal-ance in your vestibular system as well as your entire body so you feel better and are less bothered by any kind of tinnitus.

The best thing about herbal remedies is that they are gentle on the body and are still effective for tinnitus without any harmful side effects you'll see in most conventional medica-tions. Those herbal remedies used for the treatment of tinnitus support the circulation and nervous system to help the ear clear itself of excess wax and function in a balanced way so as to eliminate the excess noise in your ear.

Homeopathy Remedies

When using a homeopathic remedy for tinnitus, be sure to locate and procure the ser-vices of a skilled and practiced homeopath. Such people take special training to use herbs and other substances at specific dosage strengths to relieve symptoms that include tinnitus.

Some homeopaths use homeopathic strength salicylic acid. It is used for those who need special support, clearance and balance of their circulatory system, particularly that associated with the inner ear. The salicylic acid is taken at three times a day for two weeks or more to relieve tinnitus symptoms. Some homeopaths use salicylic acidum. It is of particular use in those who have extremely loud ringing sounds or roaring sounds, especially when the sound is associated with vertigo or deafness. It has special uses for patients with Meniere's disease as well as with those who have tinnitus caused by too much aspirin.

Calcarea carbonica can be used by those who have tinnitus alone or who have tinnitus associated with vertigo. It works best for those who have decreased hearing associated with pulsating sensations and crackling sensations in the ears. It is a good remedy for those who feel a great deal of anxiety around their tinnitus and who are easily chilled and fatigued.

Carbo vegetabilis is good for ringing in the ears associated with having the flu or with having vertigo and nausea along with it. Most of these symptoms tend to be worse at night or late in the evening. It is also associated with a special craving for fresh air. Take the dose recommended by the homeopath at three times a day for several weeks.

Cinchona officinalis is helpful if you feel anxious about sensitivity to noise or tinnitus. It is often better for tinnitus if you also have nausea, vomiting, diarrhea, sweating or blood loss. It helps replace fluids in the inner ear when you are dehydrated. It is also called "China".

Chininum sulphuricum is good for buzzing or ringing in the ears as well as having the feeling of roaring sounds in the ears that are loud enough to interfere with hearing. It also works whenever the tinnitus is associated with vertigo.

Cimicifuga is also a good treatment for tinnitus associated with noise sensitivity. It helps those who have tinnitus associated with neck and back muscle tension. People who respond well to this remedy are often too energetic and anxious about their tinnitus symptoms.

Coffea cruda is a remedy used for excitable people who are anxious about their tinnitus. It is used for the treatment of those who are sensitive about their hearing and who have a buzzing sound in the back of their head. Those who suffer from insomnia are especially well treated by this remedy.

Graphites are used in homeopathy for people who have tinnitus that is associated with deafness. It works to heal tinnitus that sounds like hissing or clicking sounds. This usually works in people who also have poor concentration as a part of their tinnitus.

Kali carbonicum is used with people who have tinnitus associated with a ringing or roaring sensation in their ears or who have crackling noises or itching in the ears. It also works well for those who have vertigo. These individuals feel their anxiety around their vertigo in their stomach.

Lycopodium is a remedy used when a person has a humming or roaring sensation in their ears along with hearing loss. It is helpful when there is an echoing in the ears or when there is a tendency toward ear infections.

Natrum salicylicum works well if the tinnitus expresses itself as a low or dull humming sound. There is usually loss of hearing associated with this tinnitus and vertigo may be present. This is a good remedy if the tinnitus is associated with influenza or with Meniere's disease.

Arnica is what's called a muscular tonic that works well for deafness and buzzing of the ears. It is used at a 30 times dilution.

Homeopathy can be difficult to explain and is not in mainstream use in the US. More mainstream doctors in Europe are using in, however, with good success. The idea behind homeopathy is to treat the person as much as one treats the disease. Many details as possible are obtained about the person and their symptoms in order to select one of many choices of homeopathic remedies used to treat the medical state. For example, the treatment of tinnitus is different if you have ringing in just one ear versus ringing in both ears.

When the symptoms are matched with the treatment, the treatment is given in dilutions of the main ingredient. Technically, the weaker the dilution, the stronger is the remedy. This flies in the face of conventional medicine and chemistry but those who use these remedies absolutely swear by the results. Even so, while little is known about how these remedies work, many people are using these remedies for tinnitus successfully. In a sense, the remedy acts like a vaccine, attempting to allow the body to heal itself.

Remedies are different for different people, even those who have similar symptoms because different people respond to remedies in different ways. It depends on a person's body type as well as on their personal preferences.

Homeopathic remedies for tinnitus are diluted to the proper dilution and are shaken or "sucussed" in water until the desired properties are achieved and small amounts (drops) of the remedy are consumed. Traditional science questions its effectiveness, indicating that the resulting remedy is much too dilute to be effective. The success of homeopathy comes from those who use it and swear by its success. Researchers on homeopathy believe that the water retains a memory of the characteristic of the diluted tincture. Clearly, much more research needs to be done to find out if homeopathy has a place in modern medicine. For those with tinnitus, however, homeopathy has many successful users so it is worth trying if you want relief.

Acupuncture and Acupressure for Tinnitus

Acupuncture and acupressure are related forms of therapy, both of which help with tinnitus. The idea is to use a needle or pressure of the fingers or thumbs to activate an energy source in your body called a "meridian". When you use acupuncture, it should be done using a certified acupuncturist. Acupressure can be done by anyone but works best when you know what meridians to activate.

Usually several needles are placed in the body and not necessarily where the problem itself is located. The acupuncturist treating tinnitus symptoms will base the symptoms on what the patient's pulse is. This determines the flow of energy in the patient's body. They will also check your tongue to know what the balance of fluid is in the body as well as the body heat. This information together helps determine what the correct treatment of the tinnitus should be.

There are several acupressure points you need to pay attention to whenever using acupressure for tinnitus. Place a single finger on the bony ridge of the skull behind the ear. The temporal bone is just above this area; it is a good point for the gallbladder. Pressure points in this area take care of the anxiety of tinnitus, headache and neck tension. Hearing loss is also treated with acupressure of the temporal bone.

Find another area in the bone just behind the earlobes. This is still the temporal bone, too, but in a different area than noted above. It is another good pressure point for tinnitus. Press on this area for several seconds to relieve tinnitus.

Another pressure point is just behind the ears on the mastoid bone and the temporal lobe above the ear lobes. This can relieve headaches, hearing loss, tinnitus and tension in the neck. This is one of the best points for relieving tinnitus, in fact.

Look at videos on YouTube or elsewhere on the web for the exact pressure points you can use. You can also ask an acupressure specialist where you can use acupressure to relieve the tinnitus symptoms.

If acupressure is too weak as a treatment, see an acupuncture specialist. Both acupuncture and acupressure are ancient Chinese remedies for various illnesses. The needles used for acupuncture are ten times as thin as needles used for medical injections. They are inserted in the meridian or energy area that represents the ears. Find a good acupuncturist or read about acupuncture in books about acupuncture so you can see a demonstration of

how it works as well as the fact that it works
for tinnitus.

The main acupuncture points your acupuncturist will use include the Yongchuan,
Taihsi, Chaohai, Taichung, Hsingchien, Yan-
glingchuan, and Tsusanli.

Reflexology

As no one knows the exact cause of many
types of tinnitus, people have turned to alternative medicine because it seems to work as
well, if not better, than traditional treatments
for this condition. One such therapy that
seems to work is reflexology. Reflexology especially works in those that have no known
cause of their tinnitus, such as those who are
younger and don't have high blood pressure
or vascular diseases. Reflexology is therapy
that works on the feet in specific areas that are
linked to body areas that are injured or sick.

One area is the base of the first three toes.
The area can be very sensitive and may hurt
when pressure is placed on it. It may take several treatments of this area, which corresponds
to the back of the neck, a common area of tension that can cause tinnitus. There are other

places on the feet that are related to tinnitus so, if you see a specialist for reflexology, you should find specific tender areas that are relieved by placing pressure on them. Many people report relief of tinnitus when reflexology is used on them. Certain foot reflexes, when triggered, correspond to the ear and can decrease the sounds of tinnitus you hear in the ears.

Tinnitus is best treated with reflexology by treating the areas involved in the liver and the kidney. These are the areas of the body involved in getting toxins out of your system. In one method of curing tinnitus, you press on the kidney and bladder area one hundred times with moderate pain. Then press the ureter area back and forth a hundred times after that. Then press the lung area back and forth a hundred times. Next, press the Yongquan, Taxi, Zhaohai, Taichong, Xingjian, Yanglingquan and Zusanli areas 30-50 times each, causing moderate pain. Finally, press the areas associated with the brain, trigeminal nerve, ear, inner ear, brainstem, liver, gallbladder, lymph nodes of the head, neck, and abdomen, the pelvic lymph nodes and the celiac plexus. Do these areas a hundred times each, causing moderate pain each time.

You can do reflexology by yourself if you know the areas to press on but, if not, a talented reflexologist is the way to go. This person can teach you how to do this yourself so you can have sustained relief of your tinnitus. It can also work on ear pain or ear infections because these conditions are related to getting tinnitus. You'll be surprised at how effective this branch of alternative medicine really is.

Aromatherapy for Tinnitus

Essential oils are very strong oils that can effectively change your mental outlook and change the way you perceive your tinnitus. It is a great therapy because it is so inexpensive and because it smells good as it is working on your tinnitus.

The essential oils best used for tinnitus are lavender, juniper and cypress oils. You can use them separately or together in a blend of essential oils. Together they help strengthen and revive bodily functions, restore the system, reduce congestion (as decongestants) and calm the nerves as sedatives. Let's take a look at these essential oils that are known to treat tinnitus.

Juniper berry is also called Juniperis communis. It carries a resinous and dry smell with deeply wooded balsamic undertones and is similar to pine fragrance. It works as a detoxifier and blood cleanser that gets rid of those toxins that might be contributing to getting tinnitus. It also helps excrete uric acid crystals and is a natural diuretic that can regulate the amount of fluid in the inner ear.

Cypress is called Cupressus sempervirens and is an essential oil squeezed out of the needles and seed cones of the cypress tree. Cypress is found near the Mediterranean Sea. It has a fresh and clean woody smell that carries a hint of spice in it that reminds one of pine oil and juniper oil.

Cypress oil is known to stimulate the circulatory system, which relieves tinnitus. It is also known to calm the nervous system—another way to relieve tinnitus. It also relieves nervous tension and stress that can make the perception of tinnitus much worse. It also helps those conditions related to the lymph system such as arthritis, sinusitis and rheumatism. In addition, it speeds healing from illness or injury.

Lavender is also known as Lavendula augustifolia. It is a distinct smell that has a spicy floral odor that is also woody and wild in nature. It is made by distilling the oil at high altitudes so as to be able to get the oil out of the flowers using lower temperatures and lower distillation pressures. This allows the more volatile phytochemicals to be intact in the distillation product.

The oil of lavender stimulates regeneration and cellular repair. It works on both the mind and body to restore damaged cells, such as the hair cells of the inner ear. It acts as a decongestion to remove excess fluid from the inner ear and gets rid of tension, stress, anxiety, palpitations and insomnia—all things that contribute to the perception of tinnitus.

How do you use these essential oils? First, you need to make an equal blend of all three essential oils (lavender, juniper and cypress) and add 15 drops of the blend to a one ounce bottle of carrier oil. Remember that essential oils are very strong and must be diluted with carrier oil. Shake the concoction well and then let it synergize for 24 hours or more.

Take one to three drops of essential oil blend to treat tinnitus by putting it on the palm of your hand and inhaling it. Put some oil on the front and back of your earlobe and on the back of the neck on the side of the tinnitus (or both sides if the tinnitus is bilateral).

Allow the oil to permeate the neurovascular system so you feel relaxed and relief from tinnitus. Don't put the oil into the ears themselves.

Make sure you use pure essential oils and not any knock-off oils. Pure oils will do the trick nicely after using it for several days or weeks. You will gradually notice a reduction in your tinnitus.

Hypnosis

Hypnosis is also called hypnotherapy or the provision of a hypnotic suggestion. It works very well for people with tinnitus, in part because it reduces stress that makes tinnitus worse. In hypnosis, you are placed in a trance-like state by a hypnotist or doctor and you are brought to a state of heightened concentration, focus and a state of inner absorption. You can concentrate on a specific word, memory, music, sound or feeling. All distraction is blocked out when you are hypnotized.

When you are placed under hypnosis, the hypnotist gives you a hypnotic suggestion, which is taken in by your mind and psyche to a greater degree because you are hypnotized.

The suggestion is used to change your behavior, sensations, perceptions and emotional state. If what you're having is therapeutic massage due to tinnitus, you should experience a decrease in the degree of tinnitus and improved hearing. This type of hypnosis is much different from the kind of hypnosis you see on the stage or on television. You maintain your free will and behavior is controlled by you—you are just able to accept a suggestion better. This translates to better health.

Make sure you use a hypnotist that specializes in medical problems and who understands the intricacies of tinnitus, how it occurs and how to manage it through hypnosis.

Chapter 6: How to Prevent Future Occurrences

Tinnitus is one disease that is better prevented than treated. Once the damage to the inner ear hair cells has occurred, it takes a lot to heal it again and many therapies are directed at coping with stress so the tinnitus fades a bit. There are few cures that completely rid you of the experience of tinnitus, whether or not you use traditional medical therapies or alternative medical therapies. What this means is that, if you have tinnitus or even if you don't have tinnitus, your focus should be on making sure it doesn't happen or making sure it does not get any worse. Ear health is important and you need to be paying attention to it.

Not always can tinnitus be prevented. In cases where the cause of tinnitus is unknown, it is difficult to say exactly how to prevent the disease from happening. Nevertheless there are simple ways to keep your ears healthy and to prevent worsening of the disease.

The single most important thing you can do to prevent tinnitus is to protect your ears from noise damage. Loud noises, heart over a long period of time can damage the hair cells and nerves in the ears. You simultaneously get hearing loss and tinnitus in the hearing frequency that your hearing loss is located in.

If you fire weapons, use loud machinery, work in industry that has loud machines, are a musician or have exposure to loud noises through the use of chain saws, you need over the ear protection. This means specialized ear protection that is far better than stuffing tissues or cotton in your ears, or even using the ear protection plugs you can get at the pharmacy. It needs to be the ear muff type of ear protection. The protection should cover for all frequencies but especially the high frequencies that seem to be more prone to damage.

If you listen to music that is amplified through an amplifier or headphones, you need to turn the volume down so that it is audible but not too loud. Even teenagers can get permanent tinnitus through the listening of music through iPods and other musical devices, including computers attached to headphones.

You can also get hearing loss when engaging in this practice. The rule of thumb is that, if others can hear the music you're listening to via headphones, the sound is too loud and you should turn it down.

Take special care of your cardiovascular health because buildup of cholesterol plaques and high blood pressure can cause tinnitus and can be perfectly well prevented through the use of regular exercise, eating foods that are low in cholesterol and fat, and taking medications if your cholesterol is naturally high due to heredity. The same is true for those who have high blood pressure because of hereditary reasons.

There are dietary things you can do to reduce the chances of getting tinnitus, primarily stopping the drinking of alcohol or cutting back on alcohol, as well as decreasing your intake of beverages that contain too much caffeine.

Smoking or even the use of smokeless tobacco products gives your body too much nicotine that, in turn, reduces the blood flow to the hearing parts of the ear by constricting the arteries and capillaries that supply these areas. This can contribute to getting tinnitus. You should stop smoking if you have already started using whatever technique works best for you and never start smoking if you are already a nonsmoker.

Exercising regularly can do wonders to prevent tinnitus. Exercise gets your blood flow moving, including the blood flow to the ears. When there is a healthy amount of blood flowing to the ears under normal pressure, the cells function better and there is a reduced chance of getting tinnitus.

Keep your weight at a healthy weight with a Body Mass Index of 25 or less. It turns out that those people with a Body Mass Index of 30 or more have a higher incidence of tinnitus. To lose weight, talk to a nutritionist about healthy ways to eat and find a trainer if you can't seem to find ways to exercise enough to lose the weight you need to lose.

Be aware that some medications will cause tinnitus. Too much aspirin, for example, will cause ringing in the ears and some antibiotics can cause permanent hearing loss and tinnitus. Ask your doctor before taking any drugs that might cause tinnitus, especially if you have some symptoms already. There are plenty of medication substitutes out there that can take the place of medications causing tinnitus.

Conclusion

Tinnitus symptoms can range from annoying to stressful to downright disabling. If you have tinnitus, it is usually something you are desperate to get rid of. Hopefully this guide has been helpful in displaying for you the reasons why you get tinnitus, what you can do to reduce the sensations felt in tinnitus, and what you can do to prevent tinnitus from happening in the first place.

As you can surmise from the reading, the ears are delicate organs with tiny bones (the malleus, incus and stapes) that can get damaged, a cochlea buried deep within the skull bones and tiny hair cells in the inner ear with hairs that can break off, get bent or get damaged completely. These hair cells are what send the signal that a sound was heard to the hearing parts of the brain. When the hair cells get damaged from excessive noise or from circulatory problems, they send random sounds to the brain and the end result is tinnitus.

When you get tinnitus, you usually perceive a sound that no one else can hear. The exception to this is certain vascular causes of tinnitus, such as having a kinked artery or vein that causes a "thrumming" sound that can be heard with a doctor's stethoscope as well as by the person with the health problem. Tinnitus can be subjective tinnitus or objective tinnitus. Most cases of tinnitus have no findable cause and are of the type of tinnitus known as "subjective" because no one else can find the cause of the tinnitus, nor can they hear it through any means.

People describe tinnitus in different ways. They can describe it as a ringing, humming, whooshing, clicking or screeching sound. Sometimes, the sound you hear can be a clue as to the cause of the tinnitus. For example, ringing sounds are often found in aspirin toxicity. Whooshing sounds can be found in certain vascular tumors or in high blood pressure as a cause of tinnitus.

Tinnitus has several different causes. It can be caused by overstimulation of sound—the constant or repetitive exposure to noise that is loud enough to damage the hair cells of the inner ear. It can be due to exposure to fire-arms, loud industrial equipment, mp3 players, other sources of loud music and chainsaws.

Tinnitus can also be caused by vascular diseases, such as kinked arteries, kinked veins, arteriovenous malformations, atherosclerosis that impedes blood flow to the ear and high blood pressure, among other things.

Finally, tinnitus can be caused by brain damage in the part of the brain that hears things. Because most tinnitus is in the elderly, however, it is most likely due to otosclerosis or vascular damage to the vessels of the ear.

Doctors may be able to hear the tinnitus in objective tinnitus but, in subjective tinnitus, doctors can use various masking techniques to assess how loud the tinnitus is. A complete physical exam is necessary to make sure that things like high blood pressure and athero-sclerosis aren't causative agents. The doctor can also use a simple scale to assess whether or not the tinnitus is loud or not.

Tinnitus, quite frankly hasn't taken up a lot of room when it comes to research on the var-ious treatments medicine has to offer those with tinnitus. This is partly because doctors don't know the cause of many cases of tinnitus and because the known causes of tinnitus are many. This means that, in traditional medicine, there are few options for treatment with the exception of some neural medications, anxiety medications and antidepressants that can make a difference in those who have tinnitus.

Some of the best ways to manage tinnitus is through alternative and natural remedies. These address several of the underlying mechanisms involved in the development of tinnitus and also address issues of stress and depression, which both play a role in how loud your tinnitus might be heard.

There are specific diets you can go on which can control tinnitus. Vegan diets and things like pineapple in your diet can improve the function of your ear. Certain exercises, including jaw exercises and general exercise can improve the tinnitus, in part by reducing blood pressure. If you have high blood pressure, you should talk to your doctor about whether diet and exercise alone can control your symptoms or if you need medication. In many instances, exercise and diet alone can control high blood pressure.

If you have access to an herbalist, choose one to help you find the right herbal remedies to treat your tinnitus. There are many herbs that have been shown to be helpful after centuries of use in the treatment of tinnitus. You can also see a homeopath for a homeopathic remedy that can be used to improve the symptoms of tinnitus using diluted essential oils and other molecules.

Some people get better from their tinnitus by means of acupuncture or acupressure. These use stimulation through needles or pressure of the energy meridians of the body using ancient Chinese techniques. They work to change the energy of the body in order to reduce symptoms of ringing in the ears by stimulating the specific meridians associated with the ear and with those areas of the body that contribute to tinnitus, such as the vascular system.

Others use reflexology to correct their tinnitus. Reflexology uses various areas on the feet that correspond to areas of the body that can help reduce tinnitus. As you have seen in the chapter involving reflexology, there are several techniques used on the feet that control the sounds heard in tinnitus.

Aromatherapy can work in some cases of tinnitus, and is inexpensive and easy to try. There are specific essential oils that work well in reducing symptoms of tinnitus.

Hypnosis can work on just about any physical ailment and tinnitus is no exception. See a qualified hypnotist to control the stress, anxiety and depression associated with tinnitus. Hypnosis can also reduce the actual sounds your ears hear.

Many doctors feel that prevention is the best way to handle tinnitus. You need to stay away from loud noises on a continual or intermittent basis, and stay away from alcohol and caffeine. It is a good idea to get into a pattern of healthy eating and exercise so your weight stays within normal limits and so you won't get tinnitus in the first place.

Made in the USA
Las Vegas, NV
17 November 2023

81044432R00046